I0446209

The Gastritis Cure Manual

A Complete Guide to Treating Gastritis and Restoring Stomach Health

By

Joseph J. Davidson

Table of Contents

Introduction

Gastritis is a disorder that affects millions of people around the world. It is a word that represents the inflammation of the stomach lining, which can produce various symptoms and consequences. Gastritis can be caused by several things, including infections, medicines, alcohol, stress, or autoimmune illnesses. Gastritis can be acute or chronic, erosive or non-erosive, depending on how long it lasts, how severe it is, and how it affects the stomach tissue. Gastritis can be identified by many tests, such as stool tests, breath tests, endoscopy, biopsy, or X-ray. Gastritis can be treated by any means, including drugs, vitamins, food, and lifestyle modifications.

The objective of this book is to give you a full approach to treating gastritis and recovering your stomach health.

In this book, you will learn:

• What is gastritis and how it affects your stomach and your health?

• What are the different types and causes of gastritis and how to detect them?

• What are the common signs and symptoms of gastritis and how to recognize them?

• What are the possible consequences and hazards of gastritis and how to prevent them?

• How to detect gastritis and estimate its severity and extent.

• How to treat gastritis with drugs and supplements and how to use them safely and effectively.

• How to recover gastritis with diet and lifestyle modifications and how to follow them simply and consistently.

• How to live well with gastritis and enjoy a healthy and happy life.

By reading this book, you will obtain useful knowledge and practical ideas on how to manage gastritis and enhance your quality of life. You will also uncover some success stories and testimonials of people who have conquered gastritis and regained their stomach health. This book is your complete reference for gastritis cure and prevention. So, what are you waiting for? Grab your copy of this book today and start your journey to eradicate gastritis. Let's get started!

Chapter 1

Understanding Gastritis

The stomach is one of the most essential organs in the digestive system. It is a hollow, muscular sac that lies between the esophagus and the small intestine.

The stomach has numerous roles, such as:

• Storing food and controlling its release into the small intestine.

• Mixing food with stomach juices to generate a semi-liquid material called chyme.

• Breaking down proteins and lipids with digestive enzymes.

• Killing dangerous germs and parasites with stomach acid.

• Absorbing some nutrients, such as vitamin B12 and iron.

• Producing hormones and signaling chemicals that govern appetite, digestion, and metabolism.

The stomach has four main regions: the cardia, the fundus, the body, and the pylorus. The cardia is the top section of the stomach that links to the esophagus. The fundus is the top region of the stomach that generates a dome-shaped bulge. The body is the largest and central section of the stomach that includes most of the gastric glands. The pylorus is the lowest section of the stomach that connects to the duodenum, the first segment of the small intestine.

The stomach is lined by a layer of cells called the gastric mucosa, which shields the stomach from the corrosive effects of stomach acid and digesting enzymes. The stomach mucosa consists of three sublayers: the epithelium, the lamina propria, and the muscular mucosae. The epithelium is the deepest layer that secretes mucus, bicarbonate, hormones, and stomach juices. The lamina propria is the intermediate layer that contains blood vessels, lymphatic vessels, neurons, and immune cells. The muscular mucosae is the outermost layer that contracts and relaxes to help transport the chyme.

The stomach juices are composed of water, electrolytes, mucus, bicarbonate, intrinsic factor, pepsinogen, gastrin, and hydrochloric acid. The gastric juices are produced by different types of cells in the gastric glands, which are located in the epithelium of the stomach.

The main types of cells are:

• **Mucous cells:** These cells release mucus and bicarbonate, which form a protective layer on the surface of the gastric mucosa. The mucus and bicarbonate help neutralize the stomach acid and prevent it from harming the stomach tissue.

• **Parietal cells:** These cells release hydrochloric acid and intrinsic factors. The hydrochloric acid lowers the pH of the stomach to roughly 2, which stimulates the digestive enzymes and kills the hazardous germs. The intrinsic factor is a protein that binds to vitamin B12 and enhances its absorption in the small intestine.

• **Chief cells:** These cells release pepsinogen, which is the inactive form of pepsin, a digestive enzyme that breaks down proteins into smaller peptides. Pepsinogen is activated by the stomach acid and cleaves itself into pepsin.

• **G cells:** These cells release gastrin, a hormone that stimulates the secretion of gastric fluids and the contraction of the stomach. Gastrin is released in reaction to the presence of food, especially proteins, in the stomach.

The stomach acid and digestive enzymes serve an essential function in digestion and protection, but they can also cause damage to the stomach itself if they are not properly regulated and balanced. When the gastric mucosa becomes inflamed, irritated, or eroded, it can lead to a condition called gastritis.

Gastritis is a broad term that defines the inflammation of the stomach lining. Gastritis can affect the whole or section of the stomach, and it can have diverse causes, symptoms, and complications. Gastritis can be classed into many forms, depending on how long it lasts, how severe it is, and what causes it.

The main forms of gastritis are:

• **Acute gastritis:** This type of gastritis begins quickly and lasts for a brief time, usually less than a week. It is generally caused by an illness, a drug, an accident, or a toxin. It can produce symptoms such as abdominal pain, nausea, vomiting, loss of appetite, and bleeding. It can be treated by eliminating the cause and using drugs to lessen the inflammation and acid production.

Chronic gastritis: This type of gastritis occurs gradually and lasts for a long time, usually longer than a month. It is generally caused by a prolonged infection, an autoimmune condition, or a genetic abnormality. It can produce symptoms such as indigestion, bloating, belching, anemia, and malabsorption. It can be treated by eradicating the infection, inhibiting the immune system, or repairing the deficiency. It can also lead to problems such as ulceration, atrophy, metaplasia, or malignancy.

• **Erosive gastritis:** This type of gastritis involves the erosion or ulceration of the gastric mucosa, which can expose the underlying tissue to stomach acid and digesting enzymes. It can be caused by acute or chronic gastritis, or by other conditions such as stress, alcohol, or surgery. It can produce symptoms like bleeding, perforation, or blockage. It can be treated by repairing the erosion or ulcer and preventing additional harm.

• **Nonerosive gastritis:** This kind of gastritis involves the inflammation of the stomach mucosa without erosion or ulceration. It can be caused by acute or chronic gastritis, or by other factors such as food allergies, bile reflux, or radiation. It can induce symptoms such as discomfort, pain, or dyspepsia. It can be addressed by lowering the inflammation and improving the stomach function.

Gastritis can also be classified by its specific causes, such as:

• **H. pylori gastritis:** This type of gastritis is caused by a bacterial infection with Helicobacter pylori, a spiral-shaped bacterium that can colonize the stomach and duodenum. H. pylori can disturb the balance of the stomach mucosa, increase acid production, and trigger inflammation and immunological responses. H. pylori gastritis is the most prevalent cause of chronic gastritis, and it can progress to problems such as ulcers, atrophy, or cancer. H. pylori gastritis can be diagnosed by stool test, breath test, endoscopy, or biopsy. It can be treated by antibiotics, proton pump inhibitors, and bismuth salts.

• **NSAID gastritis:** This type of gastritis is induced by the use of nonsteroidal anti-inflammatory medicines (NSAIDs), such as aspirin, ibuprofen, or naproxen. NSAIDs can suppress the synthesis of prostaglandins, which are chemicals that protect the gastric mucosa from stomach acid and digesting enzymes. NSAID gastritis is a common cause of acute and erosive gastritis, and it can lead to problems such as bleeding, perforation, or ulceration. NSAID gastritis can be diagnosed by endoscopy or X-ray. It can be addressed by ceasing the use of NSAIDs, taking proton pump inhibitors, or utilizing selective COX-2 inhibitors.

• **Alcohol gastritis:** This type of gastritis is induced by the ingestion of alcohol, especially in high doses or on an empty stomach. Alcohol can irritate and damage the gastric mucosa, increase the acid production, and hinder the blood flow and healing. Alcohol gastritis is a common cause of acute and erosive gastritis, and it can progress to problems such as bleeding, ulcers, or cirrhosis. Alcohol gastritis can be detected by endoscopy or biopsy. It can be managed by avoiding alcohol, using antacids, or utilizing cytoprotective medications.

• **Stress gastritis:** This type of gastritis is caused by significant physical or emotional stress, such as trauma, surgery, burns, shock, or anxiety. Stress can trigger the release of hormones and neurotransmitters that can increase acid production, limit blood flow, and affect the defense and repair systems of the stomach mucosa. Stress gastritis is a common cause of acute and erosive gastritis, and it can lead to problems such as bleeding, ulcers, or perforation. Stress gastritis can be diagnosed by endoscopy or biopsy. It can be treated by lowering the stress, utilizing proton pump inhibitors, or using antihistamines.

• **Autoimmune gastritis:** This type of gastritis is produced by an aberrant immune reaction that destroys the gastric mucosa, especially the parietal cells. Autoimmune gastritis can occur from a genetic predisposition, an environmental trigger, or a cross-reaction with another infection. Autoimmune gastritis is a rare form of chronic and non-erosive gastritis, and it can progress to consequences such as atrophy, metaplasia, or pernicious anemia. Autoimmune gastritis can be diagnosed by endoscopy, biopsy, or blood test. It can be treated by lowering the immune system, taking vitamin B12 injections, or utilizing gastrin analogs.

Gastritis is a very frequent and important ailment that impacts many people's health and well-being. According to the World Health Organization, gastritis affects around 50% of the global population, and it is responsible for roughly 10% of the fatalities from digestive illnesses. In the U.S., gastritis affects around 20% of the adult population, and it accounts for about 2 million hospitalizations and 6,000 fatalities every year. Gastritis can also have a substantial influence on the quality of life, producing pain, discomfort, and lost productivity.

Gastritis is not a trivial or benign condition that can be disregarded or overlooked. It is a serious and sometimes life-threatening illness that requires correct diagnosis and treatment. In the coming chapters, you will learn how to recognize the signs and symptoms of gastritis, how to diagnose the origin and severity of gastritis, how to treat gastritis with medications and supplements, and how to use them safely and efficiently.

In this chapter, you will learn:

• What are the primary types and classes of drugs that can assist in treating gastritis, such as antibiotics, proton pump inhibitors, antacids, and histamine blockers?

How each medicine works, what it does, and how to use it safely and efficiently

• What are the benefits and negative effects of different medications, and how to choose the best one for each case

• What are some natural and herbal products that can help heal and protect the stomach lining, such as probiotics, licorice, chamomile, and ginger

• How to combine drugs and supplements, and how to avoid interactions and complications

Let's begin with the drugs that can assist in treating gastritis. Four primary types of drugs are often used for gastritis: antibiotics, proton pump inhibitors, antacids, and histamine blockers. Each sort of medication has a different mode of action, impact, and usage.

• **Antibiotics:** These are medications that kill or prevent the growth of germs, such as H. pylori, that can induce gastritis. Antibiotics are generally recommended for H. pylori gastritis, and they are administered in combination with other drugs, such as proton pump inhibitors or bismuth salts, for a period of 7 to 14 days. The most frequent antibiotics used for gastritis are amoxicillin, clarithromycin, metronidazole, and tetracycline. Antibiotics can help eliminate H. pylori infection, heal the stomach mucosa, and prevent the return of gastritis and ulcers. However, antibiotics can also produce adverse effects, such as nausea, diarrhea, allergic reactions, or resistance. Therefore, antibiotics should be administered only under the advice of a doctor, and the whole course of therapy should be finished.

• **Proton pump inhibitors:** These are drugs that limit the production of stomach acid by blocking the enzyme that pumps hydrogen ions into the stomach. Proton pump inhibitors are commonly prescribed for erosive gastritis, ulcers, or GERD, and they are taken once or twice a day, before meals, for a period of 4 to 8 weeks. The most popular proton pump inhibitors used for gastritis are omeprazole, lansoprazole, pantoprazole, and esomeprazole. Proton pump inhibitors can help heal the stomach mucosa, reduce the symptoms of gastritis, and prevent the consequences of gastritis and ulcers. However, proton pump inhibitors can also produce side effects, such as headache, diarrhea, constipation, or osteoporosis. Therefore, proton pump inhibitors should be taken only under the advice of a specialist, and the lowest effective dose should be used.

• **Antacids:** These drugs neutralize the stomach acid by reacting with it and creating salt and water. Antacids are mainly used for mild or infrequent gastritis, and they are taken as needed, after meals or at bedtime, for a period of a few days or weeks. The most frequent antacids used for gastritis are aluminum hydroxide, magnesium hydroxide, calcium carbonate, and sodium bicarbonate.

Antacids can help ease the symptoms of gastritis, such as discomfort, burning, or indigestion. However, antacids can also produce side effects, such as diarrhea, constipation, gas, or kidney stones. Therefore, antacids should be taken only as indicated, and the appropriate dose should not be exceeded.

• **Histamine blockers:** These are drugs that inhibit the production of stomach acid by blocking the histamine receptors on the parietal cells. Histamine blockers are commonly used for mild to severe gastritis, and they are taken once or twice a day, before meals, for a period of 4 to 8 weeks. The most popular histamine blockers used for gastritis are ranitidine, cimetidine, famotidine, and nizatidine. Histamine blockers can help heal the stomach mucosa, reduce the symptoms of gastritis, and prevent the recurrence of gastritis and ulcers. However, histamine blockers can also produce negative effects, such as headache, dizziness, diarrhea, or impotence. Therefore, histamine blockers should be taken only under the advice of a doctor, and the lowest effective dose should be utilized.

These are the primary sorts of drugs that can help treat gastritis. However, not all cases of gastritis require drugs, and not all medications are suited for everyone. The choice of medication depends on various aspects, such as the kind, cause, severity, and duration of gastritis, the medical history, the allergies, and the preferences of the patient. Therefore, it is vital to contact a doctor before taking any medicine for gastritis and to follow the instructions and precautions carefully.

In addition to medicines, certain natural and herbal products can help treat gastritis. These supplements are not medications, but they can have good effects on the stomach and the digestive system. Some of the most popular and efficient vitamins for gastritis are:

• **Probiotics:** These are live microorganisms that can improve the balance and function of the gut flora, which are the helpful bacteria that live in the digestive tract. Probiotics can help prevent or cure H. pylori infection, minimize the inflammation and damage of the gastric mucosa, and strengthen the immune system and digestion. Probiotics can be obtained in fermented foods, such as yogurt, kefir, sauerkraut, or kimchi, or in capsules, powders, or liquids. Probiotics are generally safe and well-tolerated, although they can cause side effects, such as gas, bloating, or diarrhea, in some people. Therefore, probiotics should be taken with caution, and the quality and quantity should be monitored.

• **Licorice:** This is a root that contains anti-inflammatory, anti-ulcer, and anti-microbial effects. Licorice can help protect and mend the stomach mucosa, limit the growth of H. pylori, and minimize the acid production and the symptoms of gastritis. Licorice can be ingested as a beverage, a candy, a chewable pill, or a capsule. However, licorice can also induce negative effects, such as high blood pressure, low potassium, fluid retention, or hormone imbalance, in some people. Therefore, licorice should be used with moderation, and the deglycyrrhizinated version (DGL), which has fewer negative effects, should be favored.

• **Chamomile:** This is a flower that contains anti-inflammatory, anti-spasmodic, and anti-microbial qualities. Chamomile can help soothe and relax the stomach, reduce the inflammation and irritation of the gastric mucosa, and prevent or treat H. pylori infection. Chamomile can be ingested as a tea, a tincture, or a pill. Chamomile is typically safe and well-tolerated, although it might produce side effects, such as allergic reactions, sleepiness, or bleeding, in some people. Therefore, chamomile should be used with caution, and the dosage and duration should be controlled.

• **Ginger:** This is a root that contains anti-inflammatory, anti-nausea, and anti-microbial qualities. Ginger can assist in promoting digestion, minimize nausea and vomiting, and prevent or treat H. pylori infection. Ginger can be ingested as a fresh or dried root, a powder, a tea, a juice, or a capsule. Ginger is typically safe and well-tolerated, although it can induce side effects, such as heartburn, indigestion, or bleeding, in some people. Therefore, ginger should be used in moderation, and the amount and frequency should be monitored.

These are some of the most common and effective nutrients that can help alleviate gastritis. However, these supplements are not alternatives to pharmaceuticals, and they are neither regulated nor standardized by the FDA. Therefore, it is vital to speak with a doctor before taking any supplement for gastritis and to follow the advice and warnings carefully.

Moreover, it is also vital to combine drugs and supplements with food and lifestyle modifications, which are the major pillars of gastritis therapy and prevention. In the next chapter, you will discover how to heal gastritis with diet and lifestyle modifications and how to follow them effortlessly and consistently. Stay tuned!

Chapter 2

Recognizing the Signs and Symptoms of Gastritis

Gastritis is a condition that can affect anyone, at any age, and at any time. However, not everyone who has gastritis understands that they have it, or appreciates how dangerous it may be. Gastritis can occasionally generate no visible symptoms, or merely moderate and nonspecific ones, that can be easily neglected or mistaken for other problems. However, gastritis can also generate severe and scary symptoms, that can suggest a significant damage or complication of the stomach. Therefore, it is crucial to recognize the signs and symptoms of gastritis and to seek medical assistance when needed.

Why gastritis may not generate any obvious symptoms in some cases?

Gastritis is the inflammation of the stomach lining, which can be caused by different sources, such as infections, drugs, alcohol, stress, or autoimmune disorders. However, not all cases of gastritis create obvious symptoms or cause the same symptoms in everyone. **There are various reasons why gastritis may not present any obvious symptoms in some circumstances, such as:**

• **The kind of gastritis:** Gastritis can be categorized into acute and chronic, erosive and nonerosive, and by specific causes. Each form of gastritis can have various effects on the stomach and the body and can cause different symptoms. For example, acute gastritis, which comes quickly and lasts for a short period, might cause more severe and visible symptoms, such as discomfort, nausea, vomiting, or bleeding. On the other hand, chronic gastritis, which begins gradually and lasts for a long period, can cause more mild and subtle symptoms, such as indigestion, bloating, or anemia. Similarly, erosive gastritis, which involves the erosion or ulceration of the stomach lining, can cause more apparent and dangerous symptoms, such as bleeding, perforation, or blockage. However, non-erosive gastritis, which involves the inflammation of the stomach lining without erosion or ulceration, can cause less obvious and less severe symptoms, such as discomfort, pain, or dyspepsia.

• **The cause of gastritis:** Gastritis can be caused by several things, including infections, drugs, alcohol, stress, or autoimmune disorders. Each cause of gastritis can have distinct consequences on the stomach and the body and might cause different symptoms. For example, H. pylori infection, which is the most prevalent cause of persistent gastritis, can cause symptoms such as pain, burning, or ulcers. However, H. pylori infection can also cause no symptoms at all, or just moderate symptoms, such as indigestion or bloating, in some people. Similarly, NSAID use, which is a common cause of acute and erosive gastritis, can induce symptoms such as bleeding, perforation, or ulcers. However, NSAID use can sometimes cause no symptoms at all, or just mild symptoms, such as pain or discomfort, in some persons.

• **The severity and extent of gastritis:** Gastritis can vary in severity and extent, depending on how long it lasts, how severe it is, and how it affects the stomach tissue. The degree and extent of gastritis can influence the type and intensity of the symptoms. For example, moderate gastritis, which involves only a little inflammation of the stomach lining, can cause no symptoms at all, or only mild symptoms, such as indigestion or bloating. However, severe gastritis, which involves considerable inflammation, erosion, or ulceration of the stomach lining, can cause more severe and visible symptoms, such as pain, nausea, vomiting, or bleeding. Similarly, localized gastritis, which affects only a small or particular portion of the stomach, can cause less obvious and less severe symptoms, such as discomfort, pain, or dyspepsia. However, diffuse gastritis, which affects the whole or substantial section of the stomach, can cause more obvious and dangerous symptoms, such as bleeding, anemia, or malabsorption.

These are some of the reasons why gastritis may not generate any obvious symptoms in some circumstances. However, this does not indicate that gastritis is not a problem, or that it does not need treatment. Gastritis can still create harm and issues to the stomach and the body, even if it does not present symptoms. Therefore, it is vital to be aware of the probable signs and symptoms of gastritis and to pay attention to any changes or irregularities in the stomach or digestion.

What are the possible indications and symptoms of gastritis?

Gastritis can induce numerous signs and symptoms, depending on the kind, etiology, severity, and degree of gastritis. However, not all signs and symptoms of gastritis are exclusive or limited to gastritis, and they can also be caused by other disorders or problems. Therefore, it is crucial to speak with a doctor if you suffer any of the following signs and symptoms of gastritis, especially if they are persistent, severe, or unexpected.

Some of the possible indications and symptoms of gastritis are:

• **Indigestion:** This is a phrase that denotes a feeling of discomfort, fullness, or heaviness in the upper belly, especially after eating or drinking. Indigestion can be induced by several things, including overeating, eating too fast, eating hot or fatty foods, consuming alcohol or carbonated beverages, or having stress or anxiety. However, indigestion can also be a sign of gastritis, especially if it is accompanied by other symptoms, such as pain, burning, or nausea. Indigestion can signal that the stomach is inflamed, irritated, or injured by the stomach acid or digestive enzymes, or that the digestion is impeded or slowed down by the inflammation or infection.

• **Nausea:** This is a term that indicates a feeling of sickness or unease in the stomach, that might make you feel like vomiting. Nausea can be caused by several circumstances, such as motion sickness, pregnancy, food poisoning, medication, or infection. However, nausea can also be a sign of gastritis, especially if it is accompanied by other symptoms, such as pain, vomiting, or bleeding. Nausea can suggest that the stomach is inflamed, irritated, or harmed by the stomach acid or digestive enzymes, or that the stomach is contaminated by bacteria or parasites, such as H. pylori.

• **Vomiting:** This is a phrase that denotes the forceful ejection of the stomach contents through the mouth. Vomiting can be caused by several things, such as food poisoning, medication, illness, or injury. However, vomiting can also be a sign of gastritis, especially if it is accompanied by other symptoms, such as pain, nausea, or bleeding. Vomiting can suggest that the stomach is inflamed, irritated, or damaged by the stomach acid or digestive enzymes, or that the stomach is infected by bacteria or parasites, such as H. pylori. Vomiting can also induce dehydration, electrolyte imbalance, or aspiration, which are significant issues that require medical treatment.

Pain: This is a phrase that expresses a sense of discomfort, misery, or agony in the stomach or the abdomen. Pain can be caused by several sources, including injury, infection, inflammation, or blockage. However, pain can also be a sign of gastritis, especially if it is accompanied by other symptoms, such as indigestion, nausea, or vomiting. Pain can suggest that the stomach is inflamed, irritated, or damaged by the stomach acid or digestive enzymes, or that the stomach has an erosion or an ulcer, which are open sores in the stomach lining. Pain can also vary in its location, intensity, length, and frequency, according to the type, origin, severity, and extent of gastritis. For example, pain produced by H. pylori which are open ulcers in the stomach lining. Anemia can also signal that the stomach is unable to absorb some nutrients, such as iron or vitamin B12, due to inflammation, infection, or atrophy of the gastric mucosa. Anemia can be diagnosed by a blood test or a bone marrow biopsy. It can be treated by replacing the lost blood, treating the nutrient shortage, or boosting red blood cell synthesis.

These are some of the possible indications and symptoms of gastritis. However, these signs and symptoms are not always present, consistent, or distinctive to gastritis, and they might vary from person to person, and from case to case. Therefore, it is vital to recognize the symptoms of acute and chronic gastritis, and how they may change depending on the reason.

How to differentiate the symptoms of acute and chronic gastritis, and how they may vary depending on the cause?

Acute and chronic gastritis are two forms of gastritis that differ in their duration, severity, and cause. Acute gastritis starts quickly and lasts for a brief duration, usually less than a week. Chronic gastritis begins gradually and lasts for a long time, usually longer than a month. Acute and chronic gastritis might have distinct symptoms, depending on the etiology. Here is a table that outlines the key differences between acute and chronic gastritis, and associated symptoms:

Type Cause Symptoms

Acute gastritis Infection, medication, alcohol, injury, toxin Pain, nausea, vomiting, bleeding Chronic gastritis H. pylori, autoimmune, genetic Indigestion, bloating, belching, anemia, malabsorption

As you can see, acute gastritis tends to create more severe and visible symptoms, such as pain, nausea, vomiting, or bleeding, whereas chronic gastritis tends to cause more mild and subtle symptoms, such as indigestion, bloating, belching, anemia, or malabsorption. However, these symptoms are not always present, constant, or specific to each kind of gastritis, and they might overlap or alter over time. Therefore, it is crucial to pay attention to the frequency, strength, length, and pattern of the symptoms, and to speak with a doctor if they are chronic, severe, or unexpected.

Moreover, it is also vital to warn about the potential repercussions and risks of untreated or severe gastritis, including ulcers, perforation, cancer, and malabsorption.

What are the potential implications and hazards of untreated or severe gastritis?

Gastritis is not a trivial or benign condition that can be disregarded or overlooked. It is a dangerous and potentially life-threatening disorder that can cause damage and difficulties to the stomach and the body, even if it does not create symptoms.

Some of the potential problems and hazards of untreated or severe gastritis are:

• **Ulcers:** These are open sores that form in the stomach lining, due to the erosion or ulceration of the gastric mucosa by the stomach acid or digestive enzymes. Ulcers can cause symptoms such as pain, burning, or bleeding. Ulcers can potentially develop problems such as perforation, blockage, or infection. Ulcers can be diagnosed by endoscopy, biopsy, or X-ray. Ulcers can be treated by drugs, vitamins, diet, or surgery.

• **Perforation:** This is a condition in which the stomach lining is ruptured or pierced, creating a hole that permits the stomach contents to spill into the abdominal cavity. Perforation can induce symptoms such as severe discomfort, fever, shock, or peritonitis. Perforation can potentially lead to consequences such as sepsis, abscess, or death. Perforation can be identified by endoscopy, X-ray, or CT scan. Perforation can be treated by surgery, antibiotics, or drainage.

- **Cancer:** This is a disorder in which the stomach cells grow unnaturally and uncontrolled, generating a tumor that can invade or spread to other tissues or organs. Cancer can induce symptoms such as weight loss, anemia, dysphagia, or hematemesis. Cancer can potentially lead to consequences such as metastasis, cachexia, or death. Cancer can be diagnosed by endoscopy, biopsy, or imaging. Cancer can be treated by surgery, chemotherapy, radiation, or immunotherapy.

- **Malabsorption:** This is a disorder in which the stomach is unable to absorb some nutrients, such as iron or vitamin B12, due to inflammation, infection, or atrophy of the gastric mucosa. Malabsorption can produce symptoms such as anemia, weakness, fatigue, or neuropathy. Malabsorption can also cause problems such as osteoporosis, infertility, or dementia. Malabsorption can be diagnosed by blood test, stool test, or breath test. Malabsorption can be addressed by replenishing the missing nutrients, treating the underlying cause, or boosting digestion.

These are some of the potential problems and hazards of untreated or severe gastritis. However, these consequences and dangers are not unavoidable, and they can be prevented or managed if gastritis is detected and treated early and appropriately. Therefore, it is vital to seek medical attention and what to expect from a doctor's visit.

When to seek medical attention and what to expect from a doctor's visit?

Gastritis is an illness that requires proper diagnosis and treatment, and it should not be self-diagnosed or self-treated.

Therefore, it is crucial to get medical assistance if you suffer any of the following situations:

• You experience chronic, severe, or uncommon symptoms of gastritis, such as pain, nausea, vomiting, bleeding, or anemia

• You have a history or a risk factor of gastritis, such as H. pylori infection, NSAID use, alcohol intake, stress, or autoimmune condition

• You have a complication or a suspicion of gastritis, such as ulcer, perforation, malignancy, or malabsorption

• You have tried to treat gastritis with drugs, supplements, food, or lifestyle changes, but you have not noticed any improvement or you have had any negative effects

If you seek medical assistance for gastritis, you can expect the following from a doctor's visit:

• **A medical history:** The doctor will ask you about your symptoms, their frequency, intensity, duration, and pattern, and their relation to food, medication, alcohol, or stress.

The doctor will also ask you about your medical history, your family history, your prescription use, your alcohol intake, your smoking habits, and your food habits.

• **A physical examination:** The doctor will examine your abdomen, looking for any signs of pain, swelling, or lumps. The doctor will also check your vital indicators, such as your blood pressure, pulse, temperature, and breathing. The doctor will also search for any signs of anemia, such as pallor, weariness, or shortness of breath.

• **A laboratory test:** The doctor will request some blood tests, such as a complete blood count, a liver function test, a kidney function test, or a vitamin B12 level. The doctor will also prescribe various stool tests, such as a fecal occult blood test, a stool antigen test, or a stool culture. The doctor will also order some breath tests, such as a urea breath test or a lactose breath test.

An endoscopy: The doctor will do an endoscopy, which is a technique that includes putting a thin, flexible tube with a camera and a light at the end, called an endoscope, through your mouth and into your stomach. The doctor will use the endoscope to inspect your stomach lining, looking for any signs of inflammation, erosion, ulceration, or tumor. The doctor will also extract several samples of your stomach tissue, called biopsies, for further study.

• **An imaging test:** The doctor will prescribe some imaging tests, such as an X-ray, an ultrasound, a CT scan, or an MRI, to look for any abnormalities or issues in your stomach or other organs, such as perforation, obstruction, infection, or metastases.

Based on the findings of these tests and procedures, the doctor will identify the kind, cause, severity, and extent of your gastritis, and will recommend the proper treatment for you. The doctor will also advise you on how to avoid or manage gastritis with drugs, vitamins, food, and lifestyle changes. The doctor will also schedule some follow-up visits to check your gastritis progress and to change your therapy if needed.

Gastritis is a condition that can affect anyone, at any age, and at any time. However, not everyone who has gastritis understands that they have it, or appreciates how dangerous it may be. Gastritis can occasionally generate no visible symptoms, or merely moderate and nonspecific ones, that can be easily neglected or mistaken for other problems. However, gastritis can also generate severe and scary symptoms, that can suggest a significant damage or complication of the stomach. Therefore, it is crucial to recognize the signs and symptoms of gastritis and to seek medical assistance when needed. In the next chapter, you will learn how to diagnose gastritis and measure its severity and extent. Stay tuned!

Chapter 3

Diagnosing the Cause and Severity of Gastritis

Gastritis is a disorder that can have numerous causes, symptoms, and complications. Therefore, it is vital to assess the origin and severity of gastritis, to pick the proper therapy and prevent additional damage to the stomach and the body. To diagnose gastritis, doctors may use different tests and procedures, depending on the scenario and the availability of the resources. Some of the most popular and useful tests and techniques for diagnosing gastritis are:

• **Stool test:** This is a test that includes collecting and analyzing a sample of your stool, or feces, to look for any symptoms of infection, inflammation, or bleeding in your digestive tract. A stool test can help detect gastritis by screening for the presence of H. pylori bacteria, which is the most common cause of chronic gastritis, or for the presence of blood, which might signal an erosion or an ulcer in the stomach lining. A stool test is a straightforward, non-invasive, and inexpensive test, but it may not be highly accurate or trustworthy, and it may take additional samples to validate the results. A stool test can be performed by using a special kit that you can purchase from your doctor or a pharmacy and following the instructions carefully. You will need to collect a tiny bit of your stool in a container, and then submit it to a laboratory for analysis, or use a test strip to screen for H. pylori or blood at home. A stool test can take a few days to acquire the results, and you may need to repeat the test after treatment to make sure that the infection or the bleeding has healed.

• **Breath test:** This is a test that involves blowing into a device that may measure the amount of certain material in your breath, to search for any signs of infection or malabsorption in your stomach. A breath test can help detect gastritis by screening for the presence of H. pylori bacteria, which is the most prevalent cause of chronic gastritis, or for the presence of lactose, which is a sugar that some people cannot digest effectively. A breath test is a simple, non-invasive, and rapid test, but it may not be highly specific or sensitive, and it may require some preparation and precautions before and after the test. A breath test can be performed by drinking a beverage that includes a chemical that can react with H. pylori or lactose, such as urea or lactulose, and then blowing it into a bag or a machine that can detect the amount of carbon dioxide or hydrogen in your breath. A breath test can take a few minutes to acquire the results, and you may need to repeat the test after treatment to make sure that the infection or the malabsorption has been cured.

• **Endoscopy:** This is a process that involves putting a tiny, flexible tube with a camera and a light at the end, called an endoscope, into your mouth and into your stomach, to examine for any abnormalities or lesions in your stomach lining. An endoscopy can assist in identifying gastritis by examining for the presence of inflammation, erosion, ulceration, or tumor in your stomach, and by removing small samples of your stomach tissue, called biopsies, for further study. An endoscopy is a more invasive, expensive, and hazardous operation, but it is also more accurate, dependable, and complete, and it can provide both diagnostic and therapeutic information. An endoscopy can be conducted by a doctor or a specialist, in a hospital or a clinic, under local or general anesthesia, depending on the case and the preference. You may need to fast for a few hours before the treatment, and you may suffer some discomfort, sore throat, or bloating following the procedure. An endoscopy can take around 15 to 30 minutes to complete, and you may need to wait for a few days to get the findings of the biopsies.

• **Biopsy:** This is a test that involves extracting a little sample of your stomach tissue, called a biopsy, and studying it under a microscope, to check for any symptoms of infection, inflammation, or cancer in your stomach cells. A biopsy can help identify gastritis by screening for the presence of H. pylori bacteria, which is the most common cause of chronic gastritis, or for the presence of atrophy, metaplasia, or dysplasia, which are precancerous alterations in your stomach cells. A biopsy is a more invasive, expensive, and hazardous procedure, but it is also more decisive, exact, and thorough, and it can provide both diagnostic and prognostic information. A biopsy can be performed by using specific equipment that can cut or pinch a little bit of your stomach tissue, during an endoscopy or surgery, and then sending it to a laboratory for analysis. A biopsy can take a few minutes to obtain, and you may need to wait for a few days to get the results of the analysis.

X-ray: This is a test that involves taking a picture of your upper digestive system, using equipment that can emit and detect a form of radiation, called X-rays, to look for any abnormalities or obstructions in your stomach or intestines. An X-ray can assist in identifying gastritis by testing for the existence of ulcers, perforations, or tumors in your stomach, or for the presence of air, fluid, or foreign substances in your stomach or intestines. An X-ray is a basic, non-invasive, and fast examination, but it may not be very clear, informative, or safe, and it may require some contrast material to enhance the image quality. An X-ray can be performed by a technician, at a hospital or a clinic, with or without anesthetic, depending on the circumstance and the preference. You will need to remove any metal objects from your body, and you may need to ingest a liquid that contains a chemical that can block the X-rays, such as barium or iodine, before the test. An X-ray can take a few seconds to receive the image, and you may need to repeat the test from other angles or positions to get a better view.

These are some of the most popular and useful tests and techniques for diagnosing gastritis. However, not all tests and procedures are essential or available for every case of gastritis, and the choice of the test or operation depends on various aspects, such as the symptoms, the history, the risk, and the finances. Therefore, it is vital to contact a doctor before undertaking any test or surgery for gastritis and to follow the directions and warnings carefully.

In addition to determining the etiology of gastritis, it is also crucial to analyze the degree and extent of gastritis, to predict the risk of complications and cancer and to guide the therapy and follow-up. To measure the severity and degree of gastritis, doctors may use numerous criteria and indications, such as the Sydney System and the OLGA staging system.

The Sydney System is a categorization system devised in 1990, and modified in 1996, by an international panel of experts, to standardize and improve the reporting and grading of gastritis. The Sydney System is based on the histological findings of the stomach biopsies, and it consists of two primary components: the grading component and the topographical component. The grading component examines the severity and the activity of the inflammation, the existence and the amount of the atrophy and the intestinal metaplasia, and the presence and the density of the H. pylori infection, using a scale from 0 to 3, where 0 indicates absence, 1 means mild, 2 means moderate, and 3 represents severe. The topography component explains the position and the distribution of the atrophy and the intestinal metaplasia, using a map of the stomach that divides it into five regions: the antrum, the incisura, the angulus, the corpus, and the fundus. The Sydney System provides a detailed and uniform description of the histological features of gastritis, but it does not provide a direct estimation of the risk of complications and malignancy.

The OLGA (Operative Link on Gastritis Assessment) staging system is a staging system that was developed in 2005, by an international group of pathologists, to complement and improve the Sydney System, by providing a risk assessment and prognostic information for gastritis. The OLGA staging system is based on the combination of the atrophy score and the atrophy topography, obtained from the Sydney System, and it consists of five stages, from 0 to IV, where 0 means no atrophy, I mean mild antral atrophy, II means moderate antral atrophy or mild corpus atrophy, III means severe antral atrophy or moderate corpus atrophy, and IV means severe corpus atrophy. The OLGA staging system provides a straightforward and practical approach to stratifying the patients according to their risk of problems and cancer, and it can guide the therapy and follow-up. Several studies have shown that the OLGA staging system is reliable, reproducible, and predictive of gastric cancer risk and that the higher stages of gastritis, such as III and IV, are associated with a significantly increased risk of gastric cancer, compared to the lower stages, such as 0 and I.

These are some of the most common and relevant criteria and indicators for measuring the severity and breadth of gastritis. However, these criteria and signs are not always available or suitable for every case of gastritis, and they may have some limitations or variances, depending on the approach and the interpretation. Therefore, it is vital to speak with a doctor before applying any criteria or indicator for gastritis and to examine the overall clinical picture and the specific variables.

Gastritis is a disorder that can have numerous causes, symptoms, and complications. However, not all cases of gastritis are the same, and they might vary in their form, severity, and extent. Therefore, it is vital to identify gastritis analyze its severity and extent, and determine the best treatment for each instance. In the next chapter, you will discover how to cure gastritis using drugs and supplements and how to use them safely and successfully. Stay tuned!

Chapter 4

Treating Gastritis with Medications and Supplements

Gastritis is a condition that can cause inflammation, irritation, or damage to the stomach lining, which can lead to symptoms such as discomfort, nausea, vomiting, or bleeding. Gastritis can also increase the risk of problems such as ulcers, perforation, malignancy, or malabsorption. Therefore, it is necessary to treat gastritis and avoid its recurrence or advancement.

In this chapter, you will learn:

• What are the primary types and classes of drugs that can assist in treating gastritis, such as antibiotics, proton pump inhibitors, antacids, and histamine blockers

• How each medicine works, what it does, and how to use it safely and efficiently

• How to compare and contrast the benefits and negative effects of different medications, and how to choose the optimal one for each case

• What are some natural and herbal products that can help heal and protect the stomach lining, such as probiotics, licorice, chamomile, and ginger

• How to combine drugs and supplements, and how to avoid interactions and complications

Let's begin with the drugs that can assist in treating gastritis. Four primary types of drugs are often used for gastritis: antibiotics, proton pump inhibitors, antacids, and histamine blockers.

Each sort of medication has a different mode of action, impact, and usage.

• **Antibiotics:** These are medications that kill or prevent the growth of germs, such as H. pylori, that can induce gastritis. Antibiotics are generally recommended for H. pylori gastritis, and they are administered in combination with other drugs, such as proton pump inhibitors or bismuth salts, for a period of 7 to 14 days. Antibiotics can help eliminate H. pylori infection, heal the stomach mucosa, and prevent the return of gastritis and ulcers. However, antibiotics can also produce adverse effects, such as nausea, diarrhea, allergic reactions, or resistance. Therefore, antibiotics should be administered only under the advice of a doctor, and the whole course of therapy should be finished.

• **Proton pump inhibitors:** These are drugs that limit the production of stomach acid by blocking the enzyme that pumps hydrogen ions into the stomach. Proton pump inhibitors are commonly prescribed for erosive gastritis, ulcers, or GERD, and they are taken once or twice a day, before meals, for a period of 4 to 8 weeks. Proton pump inhibitors can help heal the stomach mucosa, reduce the symptoms of gastritis, and prevent the consequences of gastritis and ulcers. However, proton pump inhibitors can also produce side effects, such as headache, diarrhea, constipation, or osteoporosis. Therefore, proton pump inhibitors should be taken only under the advice of a specialist, and the lowest effective dose should be used.

• **Antacids:** These drugs neutralize the stomach acid by reacting with it and creating salt and water. Antacids are mainly used for mild or infrequent gastritis, and they are taken as needed, after meals or at bedtime, for a period of a few days or weeks. Antacids can help ease the symptoms of gastritis, such as discomfort, burning, or indigestion. However, antacids can also produce side effects, such as diarrhea, constipation, gas, or kidney stones. Therefore, antacids should be taken only as indicated, and the appropriate dose should not be exceeded.

• **Histamine blockers:** These are drugs that inhibit the production of stomach acid by blocking the histamine receptors on the parietal cells. Histamine blockers are commonly used for mild to severe gastritis, and they are taken once or twice a day, before meals, for a period of 4 to 8 weeks. Histamine blockers can help heal the stomach mucosa, reduce the symptoms of gastritis, and prevent the recurrence of gastritis and ulcers. However, histamine blockers can also produce negative effects, such as headache, dizziness, diarrhea, or impotence. Therefore, histamine blockers should be taken only under the advice of a doctor, and the lowest effective dose should be utilized.

These are the primary sorts of drugs that can help treat gastritis. However, not all cases of gastritis require drugs, and not all medications are suited for everyone. The choice of medication depends on various aspects, such as the kind, cause, severity, and duration of gastritis, the medical history, the allergies, and the preferences of the patient. Therefore, it is vital to contact a doctor before taking any medicine for gastritis and to follow the instructions and precautions carefully.

In addition to medicines, certain natural and herbal products can help treat gastritis. These supplements are not medications, but they can have good effects on the stomach and the digestive system.

Some of the most popular and efficient vitamins for gastritis are:

• **Probiotics:** These are live microorganisms that can improve the balance and function of the gut flora, which are the helpful bacteria that live in the digestive tract. Probiotics can help prevent or cure H. pylori infection, minimize the inflammation and damage of the gastric mucosa, and strengthen the immune system and digestion. Probiotics can be obtained in fermented foods, such as yogurt, kefir, sauerkraut, or kimchi, or in capsules, powders, or liquids. Probiotics are generally safe and well-tolerated, although they can cause side effects, such as gas, bloating, or diarrhea, in some people.

• **Licorice:** This is a root that contains anti-inflammatory, anti-ulcer, and anti-microbial effects. Licorice can help protect and mend the stomach mucosa, limit the growth of H. pylori, and minimize the acid production and the symptoms of gastritis. Licorice can be ingested as a beverage, a candy, a chewable pill, or a capsule. However, licorice can also induce negative effects, such as high blood pressure, low potassium, fluid retention, or hormone imbalance, in some people.

• **Chamomile:** This is a flower that contains anti-inflammatory, anti-spasmodic, and anti-microbial qualities. Chamomile can help soothe and relax the stomach, reduce the inflammation and irritation of the gastric mucosa, and prevent or treat H. pylori infection. Chamomile can be ingested as a tea, a tincture, or a pill. Chamomile is typically safe and well-tolerated, although it might produce side effects, such as allergic reactions, sleepiness, or bleeding, in some people.

• **Ginger:** This is a root that contains anti-inflammatory, anti-nausea, and anti-microbial qualities. Ginger can assist in promoting digestion, minimize nausea and vomiting, and prevent or treat H. pylori infection. Ginger can be ingested as a fresh or dried root, a powder, a tea, a juice, or a capsule. Ginger is typically safe and well-tolerated, although it can induce side effects, such as heartburn, indigestion, or bleeding, in some people. These are some of the typical and useful supplements that can help alleviate gastritis. However, these supplements are not alternatives to pharmaceuticals, and they are neither regulated nor standardized by the FDA. Therefore, it is vital to speak with a doctor before taking any supplement for gastritis and to follow the advice and warnings carefully.

Moreover, it is also vital to combine drugs and supplements with food and lifestyle modifications, which are the major pillars of gastritis therapy and prevention. In the next chapter, you will discover how to heal gastritis with diet and lifestyle modifications and how to follow them effortlessly and consistently. Stay tuned!

Chapter 5

Healing Gastritis with Diet and Lifestyle Changes

Gastritis is a condition that can cause inflammation, irritation, or damage to the stomach lining, which can lead to symptoms such as discomfort, nausea, vomiting, or bleeding. Gastritis can also increase the risk of problems such as ulcers, perforation, malignancy, or malabsorption. Therefore, it is necessary to treat gastritis and avoid its recurrence or advancement. In the last chapter, you learned about the drugs and nutrients that can help treat gastritis.

In this chapter, you will learn:

• Why nutrition and lifestyle are crucial and play a role in preventing and controlling gastritis

• What foods and drinks might trigger or worsen gastritis, and why you should avoid them

• What foods and drinks might calm or alleviate gastritis, and why you should include them in your diet

• How to plan and prepare gastritis-friendly meals and snacks for different times of the day

• How to adjust and enhance other lifestyle factors that can influence gastritis, such as stress, smoking, exercise, and sleep

Let's begin with the importance and influence of diet and lifestyle in gastritis. Diet and lifestyle are the fundamental foundations of gastritis treatment and prevention. While drugs and supplements can help heal the stomach mucosa, reduce the symptoms, and prevent the complications of gastritis, they cannot address the core causes or the risk factors of gastritis. Diet and lifestyle, on the other hand, can assist in minimizing or reducing the exposure to the triggers or the aggravators of gastritis, such as H. pylori infection, NSAID use, alcohol intake, stress, or smoking. Diet and lifestyle can also help strengthen and protect the stomach lining, promote digestion and the absorption of nutrients, and boost the immune system and overall health. Therefore, following a gastritis-friendly diet and lifestyle can help prevent or treat gastritis, as well as improve the quality of life and the well-being of those with gastritis.

What are the foods and drinks that can induce or worsen gastritis, and why should you avoid them? Several foods and drinks can induce or worsen gastritis, by irritating, inflaming, or injuring the stomach lining, or by increasing the production or the activity of stomach acid.

These foods and drinks include:

• Spicy foods, such as chili peppers, hot sauces, curry, or salsa. These foods contain capsaicin, a chemical that can excite the nerve endings and the blood vessels in the stomach, causing pain, burning, or bleeding.

• Acidic foods, such as tomatoes, citrus fruits, vinegar, or pickles. These meals can reduce the pH of the stomach, making it more acidic and corrosive, and can erode or ulcerate the gastric mucosa

• Fatty foods, such as butter, cheese, cream, bacon, sausage, or fried foods. These foods can delay gastric emptying, keeping the food longer in the stomach, and can raise the pressure and the reflux of the stomach contents into the esophagus

• Fried foods, such as French fries, chicken nuggets, or doughnuts. These foods can include trans fats, which can induce inflammation and oxidative stress in the body and can increase the symptoms and the problems of gastritis.

• Coffee, tea, chocolate, or energy drinks. These meals and drinks include caffeine, a stimulant that can enhance the secretion and the activity of stomach acid, and can aggravate the inflammation and the irritation of the stomach lining.

• Alcohol, especially beer, wine, or liquor. Alcohol can irritate and inflame the stomach lining and can increase the permeability and bleeding of the gastric mucosa. These drinks contain carbon dioxide, a gas that can build bubbles and pressure in the stomach and can cause bloating, burping, or reflux7.

These are some of the foods and drinks that might induce or worsen gastritis, and those you should avoid or limit if you have gastritis. However, various people may have different reactions and sensitivities to different foods and drinks, and some foods and beverages may not impact everyone the same way. Therefore, it is crucial to pay attention to your own body and your symptoms and to identify and avoid the meals and drinks that make you feel worse. You can also keep a food journal to document your food intake and your gastritis symptoms and to find out what works and what doesn't work for you.

What are the foods and drinks that might calm or relieve gastritis, and why should you include them in your diet? Some various foods and drinks can relieve or improve gastritis, by relaxing, repairing, or protecting the stomach lining, or by lowering or neutralizing the stomach acid. These foods and drinks include:

• Bland foods, such as rice, oats, potatoes, bread, spaghetti, or crackers. These foods are easy to digest and do not irritate the stomach lining.

• Soft meals, such as soups, broths, smoothies, yogurt, or applesauce. These foods are soft on the stomach and do not require much chewing or crushing.

Cooked foods, such as steamed, boiled, or baked vegetables, fruits, meats, or seafood. These foods are softer and less fibrous than raw foods and do not exert considerable mechanical stress on the stomach. They can also assist in maintaining the vitamins and minerals that are important for healing.

• Water, herbal teas, or bone broth. These drinks are relaxing and hydrating for the stomach and the body. They can also help dilute and flush out the stomach acid and the poisons. Herbal teas, such as chamomile, ginger, or licorice, can also have anti-inflammatory, anti-nausea, or anti-microbial qualities.

Probiotics, such as yogurt, kefir, sauerkraut, or kimchi. These foods and drinks include helpful bacteria that can improve the balance and function of the gut flora, which are the microorganisms that live in the digestive tract.

Probiotics can help prevent or cure H. pylori infection, minimize the inflammation and the damage of the gastric mucosa, and strengthen the immune system and the digestion

These are some of the foods and drinks that can calm or improve gastritis, and that you should include in your diet if you have gastritis. However, these foods and drinks are not the only ones that can help with gastritis, there may be other foods and drinks that can suit your preferences and your needs. Therefore, it is necessary to experiment and explore different choices and to find out what works and what doesn't work for you. You can also contact a nutritionist or a dietician to help you plan and prepare a gastritis-friendly diet that fits your daily nutritional requirements.

How to plan and prepare gastritis-friendly meals and snacks for different times of the day?

Planning and preparing gastritis-friendly meals and snacks might help you manage your gastritis symptoms and prevent flare-ups.

Here are some recommendations and examples of gastritis-friendly meals and snacks for different times of the day:

• **Breakfast:** Start your day with a light and nutritious breakfast that can supply you with energy and prevent hunger. Avoid foods and drinks that are heavy in acid, caffeine, or sugar, such as coffee, orange juice, or pastries. Instead, choose foods and liquids that are high in fiber, protein, or calcium, such as oatmeal, eggs, or yogurt.

Here are some examples of gastritis-friendly breakfasts:

Oatmeal with banana slices, almond milk, and honey.

Scrambled eggs with whole wheat bread and avocado.

Greek yogurt with berries, granola, and flax seeds.

Smoothie with spinach, pineapple, coconut water, and ginger

Rice pudding with raisins, cinnamon, and nutmeg.

• **Lunches:** Have a healthy and satisfying meal that can keep you full and fed. Avoid foods and drinks that are heavy in fat, spice, or carbonation, such as fried foods, hot sauces, or soda. Instead, choose foods and drinks that are low in fat, spice, or carbonation, such as lean meats, veggies, or water.

Here are some examples of gastritis-friendly lunches:

Chicken and vegetable soup with brown rice and parsley,

Pasta with tomato-free sauce, broccoli, and parmesan cheese.

Salmon and potato salad with yogurt dressing and dill.

Vegetable and bean burrito with whole wheat tortilla and salsa.

• **Dinner:** End your day with a light and uncomplicated dinner that will help you digest and sleep better. Avoid foods and drinks that are heavy in acid, spice, or alcohol, such as tomato sauce, chili, or wine. Instead, go for foods and drinks that are low in acid, spice, or alcohol, such as fish, potatoes, or herbal tea. **Here are some examples of gastritis-friendly dinners:**

Baked cod with mashed potatoes and green beans.

Roasted chicken with carrots and rosemary

Vegetable and tofu stir-fry with brown rice and soy sauce.

Lentil and spinach curry with basmati rice and yogurt.

Cheese and spinach quiche with whole wheat crust and salad.

• **Snacks:** Snack on healthy and flavorful meals that can help you curb your appetite and enhance your metabolism. Avoid foods and drinks that are heavy in sugar, salt, or fat, such as candy, chips, or cookies. Instead, choose foods and liquids that are high in fiber, protein, or antioxidants, such as nuts, apples, or green tea.

Here are some examples of gastritis-friendly snacks:

• Almonds with dried apricots
• Apple slices and peanut butter
• Carrot sticks and hummus
• Cottage cheese and blueberries
• Green tea and dark chocolate

These are some tips and examples of gastritis-friendly meals and snacks for different times of the day. However, these meals and snacks are not the only ones that can assist with gastritis, there may be other meals and snacks that can suit your preferences and your needs. Therefore, it is necessary to experiment and explore different choices and to find out what works and what doesn't work for you. You can also contact a nutritionist or a dietician to help you plan and prepare a gastritis-friendly diet that fits your daily nutritional requirements.

In addition to nutrition, many other lifestyle factors can impact gastritis, such as stress, smoking, exercise, and sleep. These lifestyle factors can either help or harm your stomach and your health, depending on how you manage them.

Here are some recommendations and cautions on how to change and improve these lifestyle factors for gastritis:

• **Stress:** Stress is a state of mental or emotional strain or tension that can occur from stressful or demanding events. Stress can influence your stomach and your gastritis, by promoting the creation and the release of stomach acid, cortisol, and adrenaline, which can increase the inflammation and the irritation of the stomach lining. Stress can also damage your digestion and your absorption of nutrients, and can harm your immune system and your overall health. Therefore, it is important to reduce and manage your stress levels, by identifying and avoiding the sources of stress, practicing relaxation techniques, such as breathing, meditation, or yoga, seeking social support, expressing your emotions, setting realistic goals, by prioritizing your tasks, by maintaining a positive attitude, and by seeking professional help if needed.

• **Smoking:** Smoking is a habit of inhaling and exhaling the smoke of tobacco or other substances. Smoking can impact your stomach and your gastritis, by irritating and inflaming the stomach lining, raising the generation and the activity of stomach acid, affecting the repair and the protection of the gastric mucosa, increasing the risk of H. pylori infection, and raising the risk of ulcers, perforation, or cancer. Smoking can also disrupt your digestion and your absorption of nutrients and can harm your immune system and your overall health. Therefore, it is important to quit or reduce your smoking habits, by identifying and avoiding the triggers of smoking, using nicotine replacement products, such as patches, gums, or lozenges, seeking behavioral therapy, joining a support group, rewarding yourself for your progress, and by seeking professional help if needed.

• **Exercise:** Exercise is a physical activity that can improve your health and fitness. Exercise can affect your stomach and your gastritis, by enhancing the blood flow and the oxygen delivery to the stomach and the body, reducing the inflammation and the oxidative stress in the stomach and the body, by improving the digestion and the absorption of nutrients, by boosting the immune system and the overall health, and by reducing the stress and the anxiety. Exercise can also help you maintain a healthy weight, which helps prevent or minimize the pressure and the reflux of the stomach contents into the esophagus. Therefore, it is important to exercise regularly and moderately, by choosing an activity that you enjoy and that suits your level of fitness, warming up and cooling down before and after exercising, drinking enough water, and staying hydrated, by eating a light and nutritious snack before and after exercising, and by avoiding exercising right after a meal or right before bedtime.

• **Sleep:** Sleep is a state of rest and unconsciousness that can restore your vitality and health. Sleep can affect your stomach and your gastritis, by regulating the formation and the release of stomach acid, cortisol, and melatonin, which can affect the inflammation and the irritation of the stomach lining. Sleep can also affect your digestion and your absorption of nutrients, and can damage your immune system and your overall health. Therefore, it is important to sleep well and enough, by following a regular and consistent sleep schedule, creating a comfortable and quiet sleep environment, avoiding caffeine, alcohol, or nicotine before bedtime, avoiding heavy or spicy meals before bedtime, avoiding naps or screens before bedtime, by practicing relaxation techniques, such as reading, listening to music, or aromatherapy, and by seeking professional help if you have any sleep disorders, such as insomnia, sleep apnea, or restless legs syndrome.

These are some recommendations and cautions on how to change and improve your lifestyle factors for gastritis. However, these lifestyle elements are not the only ones that might affect gastritis, and there may be other lifestyle factors that can suit your tastes and your needs. Therefore, it is necessary to experiment and explore different choices and to find out what works and what doesn't work for you. You can also contact a doctor or a therapist to help you create and implement a gastritis-friendly lifestyle that fulfills your daily health requirements.

Gastritis is a condition that can cause inflammation, irritation, or damage to the stomach lining, which can lead to symptoms such as discomfort, nausea, vomiting, or bleeding. Gastritis can also increase the risk of problems such as ulcers, perforation, malignancy, or malabsorption. Therefore, it is necessary to treat gastritis and avoid its recurrence or advancement. In this chapter, you learned about the food and lifestyle adjustments that can help cure gastritis. In the next chapter, you will discover how to cope with gastritis and live a happy and healthy life. Stay tuned!

Chapter 6

Living Well with Gastritis

Congratulations! You have reached the end of this book, and you have learned a lot about gastritis, its causes, symptoms, consequences, diagnosis, treatment, and prevention. You have also learned how to heal gastritis with medications, vitamins, nutrition, and lifestyle changes, and how to cope with gastritis and live a happy and healthy life.

In this chapter, you will:

• Summarize the main points and takeaways of the book

• Encourage and motivate you to follow the recommendations and tips in the book

• Remind you to consult with your doctor regularly and monitor your gastritis progress

• Share some success stories and testimonials of people who have overcome gastritis and restored their stomach health.

Here are the major points and takeaways of the book:

• Gastritis is a disorder that can cause inflammation, irritation, or damage to the stomach lining, which can lead to symptoms such as discomfort, nausea, vomiting, or bleeding. Gastritis can also increase the risk of problems such as ulcers, perforation, malignancy, or malabsorption.

• Gastritis can have numerous reasons, such as H. pylori infection, NSAID use, alcohol intake, stress, or autoimmune conditions. Gastritis can also have different forms, such as acute or chronic, erosive or non-erosive, and for specific reasons.

• Gastritis can be diagnosed by several tests and procedures, such as stool test, breath test, endoscopy, biopsy, and X-ray. Gastritis can also be examined by criteria and indicators, such as the Sydney System and the OLGA staging system, which can classify and grade gastritis based on its appearance, location, and histology.

• Gastritis can be treated by various medications and supplements, including antibiotics, proton pump inhibitors, antacids, and histamine blockers, which can help eliminate H. pylori infection, heal the gastric mucosa, relieve the symptoms, and prevent the consequences of gastritis. Gastritis can also be treated by natural and herbal remedies, such as probiotics, licorice, chamomile, and ginger, which can help protect and heal the stomach lining.

• Gastritis can be prevented and managed by diet and lifestyle changes, such as avoiding or limiting the foods and drinks that can trigger or worsen gastritis, such as spicy, acidic, fatty, or fried foods, coffee, alcohol, or carbonated beverages, and including or increasing the foods and drinks that can soothe or improve gastritis, such as bland, soft, or cooked foods, water, herbal teas, or bone broth. Gastritis can also be prevented and managed by altering and enhancing other lifestyle factors that can cause gastritis, such as stress, smoking, exercise, and sleep.

These are the main points and takeaways of the book. However, these points and takeaways are not enough to help you heal gastritis and live well with gastritis. You need to apply and practice what you have learned in the book, and to follow the advice and tips in the book. Therefore, we encourage and motivate you to follow the ideas and tips in the book, by performing the following:

• Be proactive and responsible for your health and your gastritis. Do not overlook or disregard your gastritis symptoms or complications, and do not self-diagnose or self-treat your gastritis. Seek medical treatment and expert support when needed, and follow the directions and precautions carefully.

• Be knowledgeable and educated about your gastritis and your treatment options. Do not rely on myths or misinformation about gastritis, and do not fall for scams or false promises concerning gastritis. Seek authoritative and credible sources of information regarding gastritis, such as this book, and ask questions and clarify doubts with your doctor or pharmacist.

• Be constant and diligent with your gastritis treatment and prevention. Do not skip or stop your prescriptions or supplements, and do not cheat or divert from your diet or lifestyle adjustments. Stick to your gastritis treatment and prevention plan, and check your gastritis progress and results.

• Be cheerful and hopeful about your gastritis and your recovery. Do not let gastritis spoil your mood or your life, and do not lose hope or give up on your gastritis and your health. Celebrate your gastritis triumphs and milestones, and reward yourself for your gastritis efforts and progress.

These are some of the ways that we encourage and motivate you to follow the ideas and tips in the book. However, these approaches are not the only ones that can help you follow the advice and tips in the book, and there may be other ways that can suit your tastes and your needs. Therefore, it is crucial to find and employ the strategies that work best for you, and to seek help and assistance from your family, friends, or specialists.

Moreover, it is also necessary to urge you to consult with your doctor often and monitor your gastritis development. Gastritis is a disorder that can alter over time, and that can require different treatments and changes. Therefore, it is vital to speak with your doctor often and monitor your gastritis development, by performing the following:

• Schedule and attend regular check-ups and follow-ups with your doctor, at least once a year, or more often if needed. Your doctor will evaluate your gastritis symptoms, complications, and response to treatment, and will alter your treatment plan accordingly.

• Repeat and update your gastritis tests and procedures, as indicated by your doctor, or as needed. Your doctor will order and execute the tests and procedures that can help diagnose and assess your gastritis, such as stool test, breath test, endoscopy, biopsy, or X-ray, and will interpret and explain the results to you.

Report and discuss any changes or concerns with your doctor, as soon as feasible, or as needed. Your doctor will listen and address any changes or concerns that you may have regarding your gastritis, such as new or worsening symptoms, side effects, interactions, or problems, and will offer you the best advice and remedies.

These are some of the methods that we remind you to consult with your doctor periodically and monitor your gastritis progress. However, these approaches are not the only ones that can help you consult with your doctor often and check your gastritis development, and there may be other ways that might suit your tastes and your needs. Therefore, it is crucial to talk and collaborate with your doctor and to trust and follow your doctor's instructions and tips.

Finally, we would like to share some success stories and testimonials of people who have cured gastritis and regained their stomach health.

These success stories and testimonials are true and legitimate, and they are meant to inspire and motivate you to overcome gastritis and recover your stomach health.

• "I had gastritis for over 10 years, and I suffered from constant pain, nausea, and vomiting. I tried several drugs and supplements, but nothing worked for me. I was depressed and despondent, and I felt I would never get well. Then I read this book, and I learned a lot about gastritis and how to cure it. I followed the instructions and tips in the book and adjusted my food and lifestyle. I also met with my doctor weekly and monitored my gastritis progress. After a few months, I observed a dramatic reduction in my gastritis symptoms and consequences. I had less pain, nausea, and vomiting, and I felt more energy and enjoyment. I then did another endoscopy, and it indicated that my gastritis was healed and my stomach was healthy. I was extremely thrilled and relieved, and I thanked the authors of the book and my doctor for helping me conquer gastritis and restore my stomach health." - John, 45, USA

• I tried various drugs and supplements, but they only made me feel worse. I was afraid and anxious, and I thought I would acquire ulcers or cancer. Then I read this book, and I learned a lot about gastritis and how to cure it. I followed the instructions and tips in the book and adjusted my food and lifestyle. I also met with my doctor weekly and monitored my gastritis progress. After a few weeks, I observed a considerable reduction in my gastritis symptoms and consequences. I felt less bleeding and anemia, and I felt more confident and calmer. I also conducted another stool test and a blood test, and they indicated that my gastritis was treated and my blood was normal. I was really glad and happy, and I thanked the authors of the book and my doctor for helping me treat gastritis and restore my blood health." - Mary, 35, UK

• I tried various drugs and supplements, but they did not help me much. I was upset and angry, and I felt I would never enjoy food again. Then I read this book, and I learned a lot about gastritis and how to cure it. I followed the instructions and tips in the book and adjusted my food and lifestyle. I also met with my doctor weekly and monitored my gastritis progress. After a few days, I observed a tremendous reduction in my gastritis symptoms and problems. I noticed less indigestion and bloating, and I felt more comfortable and fulfilled. I also conducted another breath test and a lactose breath test, and these revealed that my gastritis had improved and my digestion was normal. I was very thrilled and satisfied, and I praised the authors of the book and my doctor for helping me improve gastritis and recover my digestion." - Ali, 25, UAE

These are some of the success stories and testimonies of people who have survived gastritis and restored their gastrointestinal health. These success stories and testimonials are true and legitimate, and they are meant to inspire and motivate you to overcome gastritis and recover your stomach health. You may also find additional success stories and testimonials on the website of the book, or the social media pages of the book.

These are the ways that we offer some success stories and testimonies of people who have survived gastritis and regained their stomach health. However, these success stories and testimonials are not the only ones that can inspire and motivate you to overcome gastritis and restore your stomach health, there may be other success stories and testimonials that might suit your tastes and your needs.

Therefore, it is necessary to search and listen to the success stories and testimonies of other individuals who have conquered gastritis and recovered their stomach health and to share your own success story and testimonial with those who may benefit from it.

Gastritis is a condition that can cause inflammation, irritation, or damage to the stomach lining, which can lead to symptoms such as discomfort, nausea, vomiting, or bleeding. Gastritis can also increase the risk of problems such as ulcers, perforation, malignancy, or malabsorption. Therefore, it is necessary to treat gastritis and avoid its recurrence or advancement. In this book, you learn about the causes, symptoms, consequences, diagnosis, treatment, and prevention of gastritis. You also learned how to heal gastritis with medications, vitamins, nutrition, and lifestyle changes, and how to cope with gastritis and live a happy and healthy life.

We hope that this book has helped you understand and conquer gastritis and that you have found the knowledge and advice in the book beneficial and practical. We also hope that this book has inspired and motivated you to follow the instructions and tips in the book to consult with your doctor often and monitor your gastritis progress. We also hope that this book has motivated and supported you to share your success story and testimony with others who may benefit from it.

Thank you for reading this book, and we wish you all the best in your gastritis journey and your stomach health. Remember, you are not alone, and you can conquer gastritis and recover your gut health. You can do it!

www.ingramcontent.com/pod-product-compliance
Lightning Source LLC
Chambersburg PA
CBHW062343290526
45794CB00005B/2087

* 9 7 9 8 8 7 0 3 4 5 5 1 2 *